DOES SIZE REALLY MATTER?

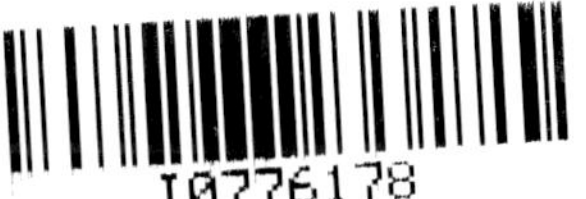

Donald Gorbach

ISBN-10 1977898033
ISBN-13 978-1977898036

"IT IS NOT THE SIZE OF A MAN BUT
THE SIZE OF HIS HEART THAT MATTERS."

—EVANDER HOLYFIELD

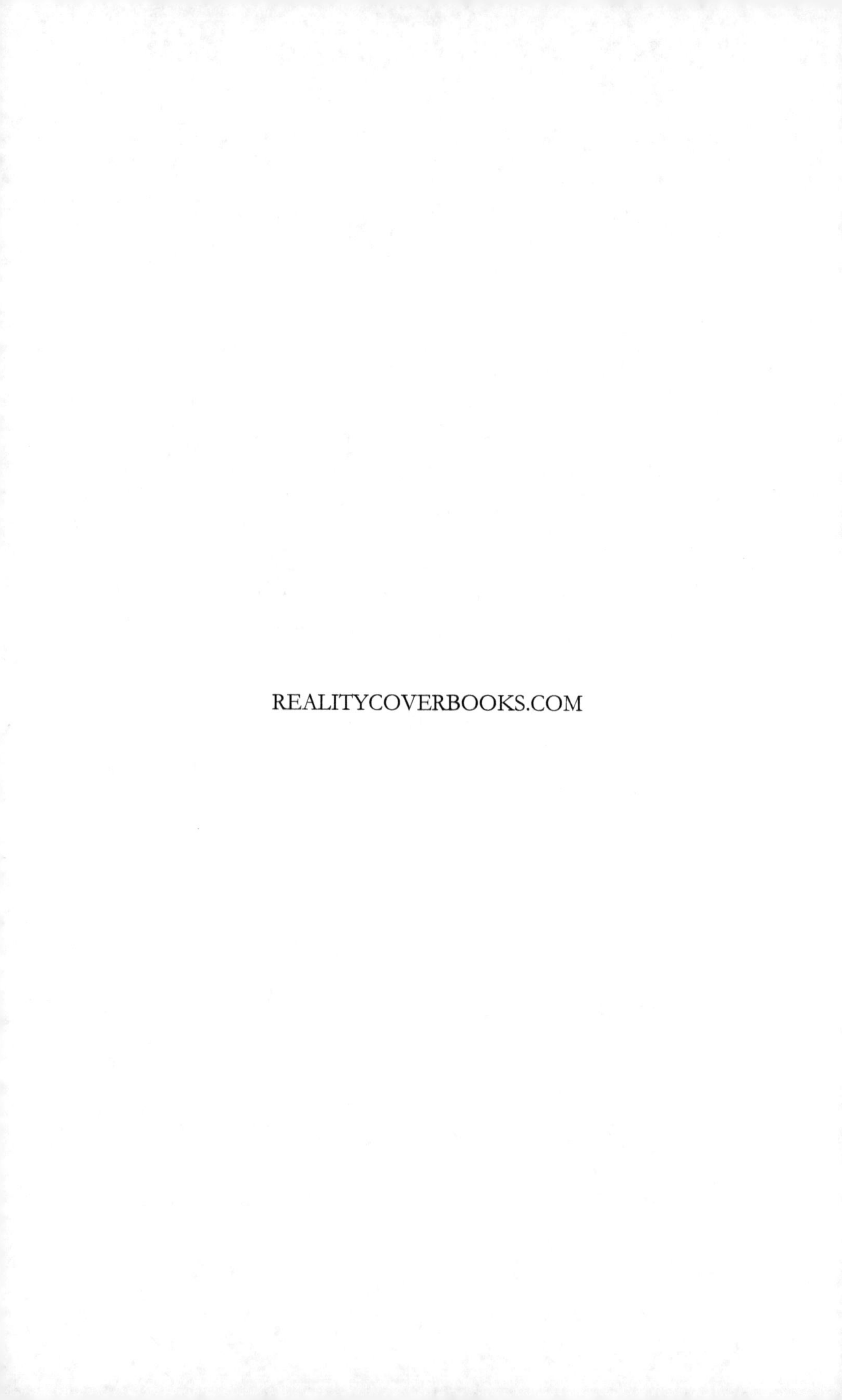